BY MSYTR
2023

NURSING AI WAR

PANORAMA ON AI APPLICATIONS IN NURSING FIELD

Nursing AI war

Msytr and Ahmed Ragab Ali Abdelghany

Published by Msytr, 2023.

While every precaution has been taken in the preparation of this book, the publisher assumes no responsibility for errors or omissions, or for damages resulting from the use of the information contained herein.

NURSING AI WAR

First edition. November 8, 2023.

Copyright © 2023 Msytr and Ahmed Ragab Ali Abdelghany.

ISBN: 979-8223670414

Written by Msytr and Ahmed Ragab Ali Abdelghany.

Artificial Intelligence Applications in Nursing:

Ahmed Ragab Ali Abdelghany "Msytr"

Table of Contents

Chapter Summaries

1. Introduction
- Introduce the concept of artificial intelligence (AI) and its growing role in healthcare.
- Discuss the significance of nursing in healthcare and how AI can enhance the nursing profession.
- Explain the structure of the book and the topics it will cover.

2. Fundamentals of Artificial Intelligence
- Define AI and explain its basic principles.
- Discuss machine learning, deep learning, and natural language processing as core AI components.
- Provide an overview of AI algorithms and tools, such as neural networks, decision trees, and reinforcement learning.

3. AI in Nursing: An Overview
- Describe the current landscape of AI applications in nursing, including the benefits and challenges.
- Discuss examples of AI-driven healthcare solutions in nursing and their impact on patient care.
- Introduce the concept of nursing informatics and its relevance to AI in nursing.

4. AI-Assisted Diagnostics
- Describe the role of AI in supporting diagnostic processes, such as image analysis and pattern recognition.
- Discuss AI applications in early detection and diagnosis of diseases, including cancer, cardiovascular disease, and infectious diseases.

- Highlight the potential of AI in improving diagnostic accuracy and reducing diagnostic errors in nursing.

5. AI in Patient Monitoring

- Explain how AI can enhance patient monitoring by analyzing data from wearable devices, sensors, and electronic health records.
- Discuss the role of AI in predicting patient deterioration and preventing adverse events.
- Highlight the potential of AI-driven remote monitoring and telehealth solutions in nursing.

6. AI-Driven Nursing Documentation

- Describe the role of AI in automating nursing documentation and reducing the administrative burden on nurses.
- Discuss AI applications in electronic health records, including natural language processing and voice recognition technologies.
- Highlight the potential benefits of AI-driven documentation, such as improved efficiency, accuracy, and patient safety.

7. AI in Nursing Education and Training

- Discuss the role of AI in enhancing nursing education and professional development through simulation, virtual reality, and adaptive learning technologies.
- Describe the potential benefits of AI-driven education, including personalized learning experiences and improved clinical reasoning skills.
- Highlight successful examples of AI-based nursing education and training programs.

8. AI in Patient Care and Support

- Explain how AI can support nurses in providing personalized, evidence-based care to patients.
- Discuss AI-driven care planning, decision support tools, and patient engagement technologies.
- Highlight the potential benefits of AI in improving patient outcomes and satisfaction.

9. Ethical Considerations

- Discuss the ethical implications of AI in nursing, including concerns about patient privacy, data security, and algorithmic bias.
- Explore the potential risks and challenges associated with AI-driven healthcare solutions, such as overreliance on technology and potential job displacement.
- Argue for the importance of ethical guidelines and responsible AI development in nursing.

10. Future Prospects: The Role of AI in Nursing
- Provide a vision for the future of AI in nursing, including potential advancements and emerging technologies.
- Discuss the potential impact of AI on nursing practice, education, and research.
- Conclude by emphasizing the importance of embracing AI in nursing while addressing its challenges and ethical considerations.

With this outline, you can begin to develop a comprehensive book on artificial intelligence applications in nursing. Remember to include references and citations to support your arguments, as well as relevant examples and case studies to illustrate the concepts you discuss. Good luck!

Introduction

Chapter 1: Introduction

1.1 The Emergence of Artificial Intelligence

Artificial Intelligence (AI) has rapidly emerged as one of the most transformative technologies of the 21st century, revolutionizing various industries and reshaping the way we live, work, and interact. AI refers to the development of computer systems that can perform tasks that typically require human intelligence, such as learning, reasoning, problem-solving, and understanding natural language. These capabilities have opened up new possibilities for innovation and growth across numerous fields, including healthcare.

In recent years, there has been a growing interest in leveraging AI to improve healthcare outcomes, reduce costs, and enhance patient experiences. This has led to the development and deployment of AI-driven solutions in various areas of healthcare, such as diagnostics, treatment planning, and patient monitoring. As a vital component of the healthcare system, the nursing profession has also begun to explore the potential benefits and implications of AI.

1.2 The Importance of Nursing in Healthcare

Nursing is a critical profession in the healthcare industry, playing a crucial role in the delivery of safe, high-quality, and patient-centered care. Nurses work on the frontlines of healthcare, providing essential services that range from health promotion and illness prevention to direct patient care and support. They are often the primary point of contact for patients and their families, acting as advocates, educators, and care coordinators.

Given the vital role that nurses play in healthcare, it is crucial to explore how AI can be harnessed to support and enhance their practice. By integrating AI-driven solutions into nursing workflows, there is potential to improve patient outcomes, increase efficiency, and reduce the burden on nurses, allowing them to focus on the core aspects of their profession.

1.3 The Intersection of AI and Nursing

The intersection of AI and nursing presents a unique opportunity to transform the future of healthcare. By leveraging AI technologies, such as machine learning, natural language processing, and computer vision, it is possible to develop innovative tools and applications that can support nurses in various aspects of their practice, such as diagnostics, patient monitoring, and care planning. Additionally, AI offers the potential to automate routine tasks, reduce administrative workload, and enhance nursing education and training.

However, the integration of AI into nursing practice also raises important ethical considerations and challenges that must be addressed. These include concerns about patient privacy, data security, and algorithmic bias, as well as the potential for overreliance on technology or job displacement. To ensure that AI is used responsibly and effectively in nursing, it is essential to engage in thoughtful discussions about these issues and develop appropriate guidelines and safeguards.

1.4 Structure of the Book

This book aims to provide a comprehensive overview of AI applications in nursing, exploring both the opportunities and challenges presented by this emerging technology. The following chapters will delve into various aspects of AI in nursing, providing insights into current trends, potential benefits, and ethical considerations.

> **Fundamentals of Artificial Intelligence** : This chapter will introduce the basic principles and concepts of AI, including machine learning, deep learning, and natural language processing, as well as key algorithms and tools.

AI in Nursing: An Overview : This chapter will provide a broad overview of AI applications in nursing, discussing the benefits, challenges, and implications of integrating AI into nursing practice.

AI-Assisted Diagnostics : This chapter will discuss the role of AI in supporting diagnostic processes, including image analysis, pattern recognition, and early detection of diseases.

AI in Patient Monitoring : This chapter will explore the potential of AI in enhancing patient monitoring, predicting patient deterioration, and preventing adverse events.

AI-Driven Nursing Documentation : This chapter will describe the role of AI in automating nursing documentation and improving the efficiency and accuracy of electronic health records.

AI in Nursing Education and Training : This chapter will discuss the potential benefits of AI-driven education and training for nurses, including personalized learning experiences and improved clinical reasoning skills.

AI in Patient Care and Support : This chapter will explore how AI can support nurses in providing personalized, evidence-based care to patients and enhancing patient engagement.

Ethical Considerations : This chapter will address the ethical implications and challenges of AI in nursing, including concerns about patient privacy, data security, and algorithmic bias, and the importance of developing ethical guidelines and safeguards.

Future Prospects: The Role of AI in Nursing : This chapter will provide a vision for the future of AI in nursing, discussing potential advancements, emerging technologies, and the impact of AI on nursing practice, education, and research.

By the end of this book, readers should have a thorough understanding of the current landscape of AI applications in nursing, as well as the potential benefits, challenges, and ethical considerations associated with this emerging technology. It is our hope that this book will inspire thoughtful discussions, encourage further research, and ultimately contribute to the responsible and effective integration of AI into nursing practice.

Fundamentals of Artificial Intelligence

Chapter 1: Fundamentals of Artificial Intelligence

Introduction

Artificial Intelligence (AI) is a rapidly evolving field that has the potential to revolutionize the way we live, work, and interact with the world around us. From self-driving cars to intelligent personal assistants, AI is becoming increasingly integrated into our daily lives. This chapter will introduce the fundamentals of AI, covering its history, key concepts, and applications.

What is Artificial Intelligence?

At its core, Artificial Intelligence is the development of computer systems that can perform tasks typically requiring human intelligence. These tasks include learning, reasoning, problem-solving, perception, and understanding natural language.

Brief History of AI

The idea of intelligent machines dates back to ancient history, with myths and stories featuring artificial beings with human-like abilities.

However, AI as a scientific field began to take shape in the mid-20th century, with the work of pioneers such as Alan Turing, John McCarthy, Marvin Minsky, and other researchers.

The 1956 Dartmouth Conference is often considered the birth of AI as a formal research discipline. The conference brought together leading scientists with the goal of exploring ways to make machines learn and think like humans. This marked the beginning of a long and ongoing journey to develop AI systems.

AI Paradigms

There are two main paradigms within AI: symbolic and connectionist. Symbolic AI, also known as "good old-fashioned AI" (GOFAI), uses symbolic representations and rule-based systems to model human intelligence. In contrast, connectionist AI focuses on neural networks and computational models that resemble the human brain's structure and function.

Symbolic AI

Symbolic AI involves creating systems that manipulate symbols and use logic to solve problems. This approach is based on the idea that human intelligence can be represented by symbols and rules for manipulating those symbols. Examples of symbolic AI include expert systems, knowledge representation, and planning algorithms.

Connectionist AI

Connectionist AI, also known as neural networks, is inspired by the human brain's structure and function. These networks consist of interconnected nodes or neurons that process and transmit information. By adjusting the connections between nodes, neural networks can learn to recognize patterns, make predictions, and solve problems. Examples of connectionist AI include deep learning, reinforcement learning, and recurrent neural networks.

AI Techniques and Algorithms

There are numerous techniques and algorithms used in AI, with some of the most important being:
1. Search and optimization algorithms
2. Machine learning
3. Logic and inference systems
4. Probabilistic reasoning
5. Planning and scheduling

6. Robotics and perception

Search and Optimization Algorithms

Search and optimization algorithms are essential to solving problems in AI. These algorithms help find optimal solutions in large search spaces, such as finding the shortest path in a graph or the best move in a game. Examples of search and optimization algorithms include A search, genetic algorithms, and hill climbing.

Machine Learning

Machine learning (ML) is a subset of AI that focuses on developing algorithms that allow computers to learn from data. ML techniques enable AI systems to improve their performance over time as they process more data. Examples of ML include supervised learning, unsupervised learning, and reinforcement learning.

Logic and Inference Systems

Logic and inference systems are used to represent and manipulate knowledge in a formal and structured way. These systems can reason, draw conclusions, and make decisions based on the given information. Examples of logic and inference systems include propositional logic, first-order logic, and fuzzy logic.

Probabilistic Reasoning

Probabilistic reasoning is a technique used to model and reason about uncertain information. It involves using probability theory to represent and manipulate uncertainty, allowing AI systems to make decisions and predictions even in the presence of incomplete or noisy data. Examples of probabilistic reasoning include Bayesian networks, Markov models, and hidden Markov models.

Planning and Scheduling

Planning and scheduling are essential AI techniques used to determine a sequence of actions that lead to achieving a goal or fulfilling a set of constraints. These techniques are widely used in domains such as logistics, manufacturing, and project management. Examples of planning and scheduling include state-space planning, hierarchical task network (HTN) planning, and constraint satisfaction problems (CSP).

Robotics and Perception

Robotics and perception enable AI systems to interact with their environment and process sensory information. Robotics involves the design and control of machines that can perform tasks autonomously or semi-autonomously. Perception focuses on interpreting sensory data, such as images and sounds, to recognize objects, analyze scenes, and understand human gestures. Examples of robotics and perception include computer vision, speech recognition, and robotic manipulation.

AI Applications

AI has numerous applications across various domains, including:

1. Healthcare: AI can assist in medical diagnosis, treatment planning, and drug discovery.

2. Finance: AI can optimizeinvestment strategies, detect fraud, and enhance customer service.

3. Transportation: AI can enable self-driving cars, optimize traffic management, and improve public transit systems.

4. Manufacturing: AI can streamline production, optimize supply chains, and enhance quality control.

5. Education: AI can personalize learning experiences, automate grading, and provide intelligent tutoring systems.

6. Entertainment: AI can create realistic virtual worlds, generate personalized content, and enhance video game experiences.

Ethics and AI

As AI becomes more integrated into our lives, ethical considerations become increasingly important. Some key ethical concerns in AI include:

1. Bias and fairness: Ensuring that AI systems do not perpetuate or exacerbate existing biases and inequalities.

2. Privacy: Balancing the use of data for AI development with individuals' right to privacy.

3. Accountability: Determining who is responsible for the actions and decisions made by AI systems.

4. Transparency: Ensuring that AI systems are understandable and explainable to users and stakeholders.

5. Job displacement: Addressing the potential job losses and social consequences of AI-driven automation.

0

AI Hardware and Software

AI systems rely on specialized hardware and software to function efficiently. Some key components include:

1. GPUs: Graphics processing units (GPUs) are essential for accelerating deep learning and other computationally-intensive AI tasks.

2. TPUs: Tensor processing units (TPUs) are custom chips designed by Google to optimize the performance of AI workloads.

3. AI frameworks: AI frameworks, such as TensorFlow and PyTorch, provide easy-to-use tools for developing and deploying AI systems

AI Terminology

To better understand AI, it is essential to be familiar with common terms and concepts:

1. Supervised learning: A type of machine learning where an AI system is trained using labeled input-output pairs.

2. Unsupervised learning: A type of machine learning where an AI system learns patterns and structures from unlabeled data.

3. Reinforcement learning: A type of machine learning where an AI system learns to make decisions by interacting with its environment and receiving feedback in the form of rewards or penalties.

4. Deep learning: A subfield of machine learning focused on neural networks with many layers, capable of learning complex representations and patterns.

5. Natural language processing (NLP): A subfield of AI focused on understanding and generating human languages.

6. Computer vision: A subfield of AI focused on processing and interpreting visual information from the world.

7. Expert systems: AI systems designed to emulate the decision-making abilities of a human expert in a specific domain.

8. Knowledge representation: Formal systems for representing and reasoning about knowledge in AI.

AI Challenges

While AI has made significant advancements, several challenges remain:

1. General AI: Developing AI systems that can perform a wide variety of tasks and adapt to new situations, similar to human intelligence.

2. Transfer learning: Enabling AI systems to apply knowledge learned in one context to new, related problems.

3. Explainable AI: Making AI systems more transparent and understandable to users and stakeholders.

4. Data scarcity: Overcoming the limitations imposed by insufficient or unrepresentative data.

Future of AI

The future of AI is filled with potential, and the field is expected to continue to grow and evolve rapidly. Some key areas of future AI research and development include:

1. Neuromorphic computing: Developing hardware and software that more closely mimics the structure and function of the human brain.

2. AI safety: Ensuring that AI systems are designed and deployed in a way that minimizes risks and unintended consequences.

3. Human-AI collaboration: Enhancing the interaction between humans and AI systems to enable more effective and efficient cooperation.

4. AI policy and regulation: Developing policies and regulations to govern the development and use of AI technolog

Conclusion

Artificial Intelligence is a complex and multidisciplinary field that seeks to create intelligent machines capable of performing tasks that typically require human intelligence. By understanding the fundamentals of AI, including its history, key concepts, and applications, you can better appreciate the potential this technology holds for transforming our world and shaping our future. As AI continues to advance, it is essential to remain informed about its progress and engage in discussions about its ethical implications and societal impact.

AI in Nursing: An Overview

Chapter 2: AI in Nursing: An Overview
Introduction

The integration of Artificial Intelligence (AI) into healthcare has the potential to transform the way medical professionals work and deliver care to patients. One area where AI can have a significant impact is nursing, as it can help streamline workflows, improve patient outcomes, and empower nurses to make better-informed decisions. This chapter will provide an overview of AI in nursing, discussing its applications, benefits, challenges, and future prospects.

AI in Nursing: Why It Matters

Nursing is a critical component of healthcare, responsible for providing patient care, education, and support. As the demand for healthcare services continues to rise, nurses face increasing workloads and pressure to deliver high-quality care. AI can help alleviate some of this burden by automating routine tasks, providing decision support, and enabling more effective communication.

Applications of AI in Nursing

AI can be applied to various aspects of nursing, including:
1. Patient triage and assessment
2. Care planning and coordination
3. Medication management
4. Remote monitoring and telehealth
5. Workflow optimization
6. Education and training

Patient Triage and Assessment

AI can support nurses in triaging patients and assessing their condition. For example, natural language processing (NLP) algorithms can analyze patient records, identify relevant information, and suggest a priority level for care. AI can also assist in evaluating patients' vital signs and detecting early warning signs of deterioration, allowing nurses to intervene promptly.

Care Planning and Coordination

AI can help nurses develop personalized care plans by analyzing patient data, identifying potential risks, and recommending evidence-based interventions. Additionally, AI can support care coordination by facilitating communication between different healthcare providers and ensuring that all relevant information is readily available.

Medication Management

AI can play a crucial role in medication management, helping to prevent medication errors and ensure patient safety. For example, AI algorithms can analyze patient data to identify potential drug interactions, allergies, or contraindications. AI can also assist in monitoring patients' adherence to medication regimens and provide reminders for medication administration.

Remote Monitoring and Telehealth

AI can enhance remote monitoring and telehealth services by analyzing data from wearable devices, mobile apps, and home monitoring equipment. This allows nurses to track patients' health status, detect potential issues, and intervene appropriately. Telehealth services can also incorporate AI-powered virtual nursing assistants that can answer patients' questions, provide health advice, and escalate concerns when necessary.

Workflow Optimization

AI can help optimize nursing workflows by automating routine tasks, such as documentation and data entry, freeing up time for nurses to focus on patient care. Additionally, AI can support nurses in managing their schedules, prioritizing tasks, and allocating resources more effectively.

Education and Training

AI can enhance nursing education and training by providing personalized learning experiences, simulating real-world scenarios, and offering real-time feedback. For example, AI-powered virtual reality (VR) and augmented reality (AR) environments can allow nurses to practice skills and procedures in a safe, interactive setting.

Benefits of AI in Nursing

The integration of AI into nursing can offer several benefits, including:

1. Improved patient outcomes
2. Enhanced decision-making
3. Increased efficiency and cost savings
4. Better communication and collaboration

Improved Patient Outcomes

By providing decision support, automating routine tasks, and enabling early intervention, AI can help nurses deliver more effective and timely care, ultimately improving patient outcomes. For instance, AI-powered early warning systems can help detect sepsis or other complications, allowing for prompt treatment and potentially saving lives.

Enhanced Decision-Making

AI can support nurses in making better-informed decisions by providing access to relevant, up-to-date information and evidence-based recommendations. This can help ensure that patients receive the most appropriate care and minimize the risk of adverse events or complications.

Increased Efficiency and Cost Savings

By streamlining workflows and automating time-consuming tasks, AI can help increase efficiency and reduce costs in nursing. For example, AI-powered documentation systems can reduce the time nurses spend on paperwork, allowing them to devote more time to patient care and reducing the risk of burnout.

Better Communication and Collaboration

AI can facilitate communication and collaboration between nurses and other healthcare professionals, ensuring that all team members have access to the information they need to provide coordinated, high-quality care. For example, AI-powered care coordination platforms can help manage patient handoffs, minimize communication gaps, and enable seamless information sharing.

Challenges and Barriers to AI Adoption in Nursing

While AI holds great promise for nursing, several challenges and barriers must be addressed for its successful implementation, including:

1. Data quality and availability
2. Integration with existing systems
3. Legal and ethical considerations
4. Workforce training and acceptance

Data Quality and Availability

AI algorithms rely onlarge volumes of high-quality data to function effectively. However, healthcare data can be fragmented, incomplete, or inconsistent, making it challenging to develop and implement AI systems. Ensuring data quality and interoperability is essential for the successful integration of AI into nursing.

Integration with Existing Systems

Integrating AI technologies into existing healthcare systems can be complex and time-consuming. Organizations must carefully consider how AI tools will interact with current electronic health record (HER) systems, workflow management solutions, and other technologies. Additionally, ensuring compatibility and seamless information sharing between different systems is critical.

Legal and Ethical Considerations

The use of AI in nursing raises several legal and ethical questions, such as data privacy, security, and accountability. Healthcare organizations must ensure that AI systems comply with relevant regulations, protect patient confidentiality, and maintain transparency in decision-making processes.

Workforce Training and Acceptance

For AI to be effective in nursing, the workforce must be trained to use these new technologies and accept them as part of their daily practice. This requires ongoing education, support, and change management efforts to help nurses understand the benefits of AI and overcome any fears or misconceptions.

The Future of AI in Nursing

As AI technologies continue to evolve, the potential applications and benefits for nursing will only increase. Some key areas of future development include:

1. Personalized and precision nursing
2. Enhanced patient engagement
3. AI-assisted robotics in nursing
4. Advanced predictive analytics

Personalized and Precision Nursing

AI has the potential to enable a more personalized and precise approach to nursing, tailoring care plans to each patient's unique needs and circumstances. By analyzing large volumes of data, AI algorithms can identify patterns and associations that can inform care decisions and help predict patient outcomes.

Enhanced Patient Engagement

AI can also play a role in improving patient engagement by providing personalized health information, recommendations, and support through digital platforms and virtual nursing assistants. This can help patients take a more active role in their care, leading to better outcomes and increased satisfaction.

AI-Assisted Robotics in Nursing

Robotic technology, powered by AI, can offer valuable support in various nursing tasks, such as medication administration, patient lifting, and mobility assistance. As AI and robotic technologies continue to advance, the potential for AI-assisted robotics in nursing will only grow.

Advanced Predictive Analytics

AI's ability to analyze vast amounts of data can enable advanced predictive analytics in nursing. This can help identify patients at risk for complications or readmissions, allowing for early intervention and potentially improving patient outcomes.

Conclusion

AI holds significant potential to transform nursing and improve patient care. By harnessing the power of AI, nurses can access better decision support, streamline workflows, and deliver more personalized, effective care. However, successful integration of AI into nursing will require addressing challenges such as data quality, workforce training, and ethical considerations.

As AI technologies continue to evolve, the future of nursing is poised to become increasingly data-driven and technologically advanced. Embracing AI and its potential applications in nursing can help healthcare organizations and professionals deliver high-quality care, improve patient outcomes, and navigate the challenges of an ever-evolving healthcare landscape.

AI-Assisted Diagnosis: A Comprehensive Overview

Chapter 3: AI-Assisted Diagnosis: A Comprehensive Overvie.

Introduction

The rise of artificial intelligence (AI) in healthcare has opened the door to a new era of AI-assisted diagnosis, which has the potential to revolutionize the way medical professionals diagnose and treat various medical conditions. By harnessing the power of AI, clinicians can improve diagnostic accuracy, reduce diagnostic errors, and streamline workflows. This chapter will provide a comprehensive overview of AI-assisted diagnosis, covering its applications, benefits, challenges, and future prospects.

The Role of AI in Diagnosis

Diagnosis is a critical step in the healthcare process, as it informs subsequent treatment decisions and can significantly impact patient outcomes. AI can play a key role in enhancing the diagnostic process by providing decision support, automating complex tasks, and enabling more effective use of medical data.

Applications of AI-Assisted Diagnosis

AI-assisted diagnosis can be applied to a wide range of medical fields, including:

1. Radiology and medical imaging
2. Pathology
3. Dermatology
4. Ophthalmology

5. Cardiology

6. Oncology

Radiology and Medical Imaging

AI has made significant strides in the field of radiology and medical imaging. AI algorithms, particularly deep learning-based models such as convolutional neural networks (CNNs), have shown great promise in detecting and diagnosing various conditions from medical images, including tumors, fractures, and lung abnormalities.

For instance, AI systems can be trained to analyze X-rays, CT scans, and MRI images, identifying patterns and abnormalities that may be indicative of a specific condition. These systems can then provide diagnostic suggestions to radiologists, improving accuracy and reducing the time needed to interpret images.

Pathology

AI-assisted diagnosis is also making an impact in pathology, where AI algorithms can analyze digital pathology slides and identify cellular or molecular markers associated with various diseases. This can help pathologists make more accurate diagnoses, particularly in complex cases where subtle differences between conditions may be challenging to discern.

Dermatology

In dermatology, AI systems can be used to analyze images of skin lesions and provide diagnostic suggestions for conditions such as skin cancer, psoriasis, and eczema. By comparing the characteristics of a patient's lesion to a database of known conditions, AI algorithms can help dermatologists make more accurate and timely diagnoses.

Ophthalmology

AI-assisted diagnosis has potential applications in ophthalmology, where AI algorithms can analyze retinal images and detect signs of various eye diseases, such as diabetic retinopathy, age-related macular degeneration, and glaucoma. Early detection and diagnosis of these conditions can be crucial in preventing vision loss and improving patient outcomes.

Cardiology

In cardiology, AI systems can be used to analyze electrocardiogram (ECG) data, detect arrhythmias, and assess cardiac function. AI algorithms can help cardiologists interpret complex ECG patterns, identify potential risks, and make more informed treatment decisions.

Oncology

AI-assisted diagnosis is also being explored in oncology, where AI algorithms can analyze various types of medical data, such as imaging studies, genomic data, and clinical information, to identify potential cancerous lesions and predict treatment response. This can help oncologists make more accurate and personalized treatment decisions for their patients.

Benefits of AI-Assisted Diagnosis

The integration of AI into the diagnostic process offers several benefits, including:

1. Improved diagnostic accuracy
2. Reduced diagnostic errors
3. Streamlined workflows
4. Enhanced collaboration and decision support

Improved Diagnostic Accuracy

One of the primary benefits of AI-assisted diagnosis is the potential for improved diagnostic accuracy. By analyzing large volumes of data and identifying patterns and associations that may be difficult for human clinicians to discern, AI algorithms can help healthcare professionals make more accurate diagnoses and ultimately improve patient outcomes.

Reduced Diagnostic Errors

Diagnostic errors can have significant consequences for patients, leading to incorrect or delayed treatment and potentially worsening outcomes. AI-assisted diagnosis can help reduce the risk of diagnostic errors by providing decision support, automating complex tasks, and enabling more effective use of medical data.

Streamlined Workflows

AI can help streamline diagnostic workflows by automating time-consuming tasks, such as analyzing medical images or processing laboratory data. This can free up time for healthcare professionals to focus on patient care and reduce the risk of burnout.

Enhanced Collaboration and Decision Support

AI-assisted diagnosis can facilitate collaboration between healthcare professionals by providing a shared platform for data analysis and decision-making. This can help ensure that all team members have access to the information they need to provide coordinated, high-quality care.

Challenges and Barriers to AI-Assisted Diagnosis

Despite the promising potential of AI-assisted diagnosis, several challenges and barriers must be addressed for its successful implementation, including:

1. Data quality and availability
2. Integration

Integration with Existing Systems

Integrating AI-assisted diagnosis into existing healthcare systems can be a complex process, requiring the coordination of various stakeholders, including medical professionals, IT teams, and administrators. Ensuring seamless integration with existing workflows, electronic health records (EHRs), and other clinical systems is essential for maximizing the benefits of AI in diagnosis.

Algorithmic Bias and Fairness

AI algorithms are trained on large datasets, and the quality of these datasets can directly impact the performance and fairness of AI-assisted diagnosis systems. If the training data is biased or unrepresentative, the AI system may perpetuate existing biases and contribute to health disparities. Ensuring that AI algorithms are trained on diverse and representative datasets is critical for promoting fair and equitable healthcare outcomes.

Regulatory and Ethical Considerations

AI-assisted diagnosis raises various regulatory and ethical concerns, including issues related to patient privacy, data security, and algorithmic transparency. Navigating the complex regulatory landscape and ensuring compliance with applicable laws and ethical guidelines is essential for the successful implementation of AI in healthcare.

User Acceptance and Trust

Building trust and acceptance among healthcare professionals and patients is another challenge for AI-assisted diagnosis. Ensuring that AI systems are transparent, reliable, and user-friendly is crucial for fostering trust and promoting adoption among clinicians and patients alike.

The Future of AI-Assisted Diagnosis

As AI technologies continue to advance, the potential applications and benefits of AI-assisted diagnosis are expected to grow. Future developments in AI-assisted diagnosis may include:

1. Personalized medicine
2. Predictive analytics and risk stratification
3. Integration with telemedicine
4. Expansion to underserved communities

Personalized Medicine

By leveraging the power of AI, healthcare professionals will be better equipped to provide personalized medicine, tailoring treatment plans based on each patient's unique genetic, environmental, and lifestyle factors. AI-assisted diagnosis can help identify specific biomarkers and predict treatment response, enabling more targeted and effective therapeutic interventions.

Predictive Analytics and Risk Stratification

AI-assisted diagnosis can also be used to predict patient outcomes and stratify risk, helping healthcare professionals identify high-risk individuals and target interventions accordingly. This can help optimize resource allocation and improve the overall efficiency of healthcare delivery.

Integration with Telemedicine

As telemedicine becomes increasingly prevalent, AI-assisted diagnosis can be integrated into virtual care platforms, enabling remote diagnosis and expanding access to specialized care for patients in rural or underserved communities.

Expansion to Underserved Communities

AI-assisted diagnosis has the potential to bridge gaps in healthcare access and quality, particularly in underserved communities. By enabling remote diagnosis and facilitating collaboration between healthcare professionals, AI can help ensure that all patients have access to high-quality care, regardless of their geographic location or socioeconomic status.

Conclusion

AI-assisted diagnosis is poised to revolutionize the way medical professionals diagnose and treat various medical conditions. By harnessing the power of AI, healthcare professionals can improve diagnostic accuracy, reduce diagnostic errors, and streamline workflows. While challenges and barriers remain, the future of AI-assisted diagnosis holds great promise for enhancing patient care and outcomes.

AI in Patient Monitoring: A Comprehensive Overview

Chapter 4: AI in Patient Monitoring: A Comprehensive Overview

Introduction

Artificial intelligence (AI) is transforming the healthcare landscape, and one of the most promising areas of application is patient monitoring. AI-powered patient monitoring systems can analyze large volumes of data in real-time, providing healthcare professionals with critical insights that can guide care decisions and improve patient outcomes. This chapter will provide a comprehensive overview of AI in patient monitoring, covering its applications, benefits, challenges, and future prospects.

The Role of AI in Patient Monitoring

Patient monitoring is a key aspect of healthcare, allowing clinicians to track a patient's vital signs, symptoms, and other health indicators over time. AI can enhance patient monitoring by automating the analysis of complex datasets, identifying patterns and trends that may be difficult for human clinicians to discern, and providing real-time alerts and decision support.

Applications of AI in Patient Monitoring

AI-powered patient monitoring systems can be applied to a wide range of healthcare settings, including:

1. Intensive care units (ICUs)

2. Emergency departments

3. Inpatient wards

4. Remote and home-based monitoring

Intensive Care Units (ICUs)

In the ICU, the stakes are high, and patient conditions can change rapidly. AI-powered monitoring systems can provide continuous, real-time analysis of vital signs and other clinical data, helping to identify early warning signs of patient deterioration and enabling timely interventions.

For instance, AI algorithms can analyze physiological data, such as heart rate, blood pressure, and oxygen saturation, to detect patterns indicative of sepsis, acute kidney injury, or other life-threatening conditions. By providing real-time alerts, AI can help clinicians intervene more quickly, potentially improving patient outcomes.

Emergency Departments

In emergency departments, timely and accurate triage is critical for optimizing patient outcomes. AI-powered monitoring systems can assist with triage by analyzing vital signs, chief complaints, and other clinical data to prioritize patients based on their risk of deterioration.

For example, AI algorithms can be used to predict the likelihood of a patient experiencing a cardiac event, allowing clinicians to prioritize care for those at highest risk. This can help ensure that resources are allocated effectively and that high-risk patients receive the care they need without delay.

Inpatient Wards

On inpatient wards, AI-powered patient monitoring systems can support clinical decision-making by providing continuous analysis of patient data and identifying trends that may warrant further investigation. This can help healthcare professionals detect early signs of complications, such as infections or adverse drug reactions, and intervene as needed to optimize patient outcomes.

Remote and Home-Based Monitoring

As telehealth and home-based care become increasingly prevalent, AI-powered patient monitoring systems have significant potential to enhance remote care delivery. By analyzing data from wearable devices and other remote monitoring tools, AI algorithms can provide real-time insights into patient health, enabling early intervention and more responsive care.

Benefits of AI in Patient Monitoring

The integration of AI into patient monitoring offers several benefits, including:

1. Improved patient outcomes
2. Enhanced clinical decision support
3. Streamlined workflows
4. Reduced healthcare costs

Improved Patient Outcomes

One of the primary benefits of AI-powered patient monitoring is the potential for improved patient outcomes. By providing real-time analysis of patient data and alerting clinicians to early warning signs of deterioration, AI can help ensure that patients receive timely and appropriate interventions, ultimately improving their chances of recovery.

Enhanced Clinical Decision Support

AI can also provide valuable decision support for healthcare professionals, helping them identify patterns and trends in patient data that may warrant further investigation or intervention. This can help clinicians make more informed decisions about patient care and ensure that resources are allocated effectively.

Streamlined Workflows

AI-powered patient monitoring systems can help streamline clinical workflows by automating the analysis of patient data, reducing the cognitive burden on healthcare professionals, and freeing up time for direct patient care. This can help improve the overall efficiency of healthcare delivery and reduce the risk of clinician burnout.

Reduced Healthcare Costs

By improving patient outcomes, streamlining workflows, and optimizing resource allocation, AI-powered patient monitoring systems have the potential to reduce healthcare costs. This can make healthcare more accessible and affordable for patients and help ensure the sustainability of healthcare systems.

Challenges and Barriers to AI in Patient Monitoring

Despite the promising potential of AI in patient monitoring, several challenges and barriers must be addressed for its successful implementation, including:

1. Data quality and availability
2. Integration with existing systems
3. Regulatory and ethical considerations
4. User acceptance and trust

Data Quality and Availability

The success of AI-powered patient monitoring is heavily dependent on the quality and availability of patient data. Ensuring that data is accurate, complete, and representative is critical for training AI algorithms and ensuring their reliable performance.

Integration with Existing Systems

Integrating AI-powered patient monitoringsystems with existing healthcare infrastructure can be challenging. Interoperability between different electronic health record (EHR) systems, monitoring devices, and data formats is essential for seamless integration and effective data exchange.

Regulatory and Ethical Considerations

The use of AI in patient monitoring raises several regulatory and ethical concerns, including data privacy, informed consent, and algorithmic bias. Ensuring that AI systems are transparent, accountable, and adhere to relevant regulations and ethical guidelines is crucial for their successful implementation.

User Acceptance and Trust

For AI-powered patient monitoring systems to be successful, healthcare professionals and patients must trust and accept the technology. This requires addressing concerns around the accuracy and reliability of AI algorithms, as well as providing adequate training and support for healthcare professionals using the technology.

Future Prospects of AI in Patient Monitoring

The future of AI in patient monitoring is promising, with several areas of potential growth and advancement, including:

1. Personalized medicine
2. Predictive analytics
3. Integration of multimodal data
4. Augmented reality and virtual reality

Personalized Medicine

AI-powered patient monitoring systems have the potential to support personalized medicine by providing tailored care recommendations based on individual patient characteristics and needs.

For example, AI algorithms could analyze genetic, environmental, and lifestyle factors to predict a patient's risk of developing certain conditions or experiencing adverse drug reactions. This information could be used to guide personalized care plans, optimize treatment strategies, and improve patient outcomes.

Predictive Analytics

AI has the potential to shift the focus of patient monitoring from reactive to proactive care by using predictive analytics to identify patients at risk of future health events or complications.

For instance, AI algorithms could analyze historical and real-time patient data to predict the likelihood of readmission, the development of chronic conditions, or the need for hospitalization. These insights could be used to guide preventive interventions, such as lifestyle modifications or medication adjustments, and ultimately improve patient outcomes.

Integration of Multimodal Data

The integration of multimodal data, such as medical imaging, electronic health records, and wearable device data, can provide a more comprehensive view of patient health and enhance the accuracy and reliability of AI-powered patient monitoring systems.

For example, AI algorithms could analyze data from multiple sources to predict the progression of diseases like Alzheimer's or Parkinson's, enabling more proactive and targeted interventions to slow down disease progression and improve quality of life.

Augmented Reality and Virtual Reality

Augmented reality (AR) and virtual reality (VR) technologies have the potential to revolutionize patient monitoring by providing immersive, interactive, and real-time visualizations of patient data.

For instance, AR headsets could display real-time patient vital signs, alerts, and decision support information directly in a clinician's field of view, reducing the need for constant monitoring of screens and devices. Similarly, VR simulations could be used for training and education purposes, helping healthcare professionals develop the skills needed to effectively use AI-powered patient monitoring systems.

Conclusion

AI-powered patient monitoring systems hold significant promise for enhancing healthcare delivery and improving patient outcomes. By providing real-time analysis of patient data, identifying early warning signs of deterioration, and offering decision support, AI has the potential to revolutionize patient monitoring and transform the healthcare landscape.

However, several challenges and barriers must be addressed for the successful implementation of AI in patient monitoring, including data quality and availability, integration with existing systems, regulatory and ethical considerations, and user acceptance and trust.

Looking to the future, advancements in personalized medicine, predictive analytics, multimodal data integration, and AR/VR technologies offer exciting opportunities for the further development and application of AI in patient monitoring. As the capabilities of AI continue to expand, its impact on patient monitoring and healthcare more broadly is likely to grow, offering new possibilities for the enhancement of patient care and the optimization of healthcare delivery.

AI-Driven Nursing Documentation: A Comprehensive Overview

Chapter 7: AI-Driven Nursing Documentation: A Comprehensive Overview

Introduction

Artificial intelligence (AI) is revolutionizing various aspects of healthcare, and one of the key areas of application is nursing documentation. Efficient and accurate nursing documentation is crucial for maintaining high-quality patient care and ensuring effective communication among healthcare professionals. AI-driven nursing documentation can streamline the documentation process, reduce errors, and improve the overall quality of patient records. This chapter will provide an in-depth overview of AI in nursing documentation, covering its applications, benefits, challenges, and future prospects.

The Role of AI in Nursing Documentation

Nursing documentation is an essential component of patient care, serving as a means of communication among healthcare professionals and providing a record of the care provided. AI can enhance nursing documentation by automating the generation, organization, and analysis of patient records, reducing the burden on nursing staff and improving the quality of the documentation.

Applications of AI in Nursing Documentation

AI-driven nursing documentation can be applied in various ways to improve the efficiency and accuracy of nursing documentation, including:

1. Natural language processing (NLP) and generation
2. Voice recognition and transcription
3. Computer vision and image recognition
4. Predictive analytics for care planning

Natural Language Processing (NLP) and Generation

NLP techniques can be used to analyze and interpret free-text nursing notes, identifying key information and organizing it into structured formats. This can help streamline the documentation process and improve the consistency and accuracy of patient records.

Moreover, AI-driven natural language generation (NLG) can be used to automatically generate nursing notes based on structured data inputs, reducing the time and effort required for manual documentation.

Voice Recognition and Transcription

AI-powered voice recognition and transcription technologies can enable nursing staff to dictate their notes verbally, with the AI system transcribing the speech into written text. This can help reduce the time spent on documentation and minimize typing errors, improving the overall efficiency and accuracy of nursing documentation.

Computer Vision and Image Recognition

AI-driven computer vision and image recognition technologies can be used to analyze and interpret medical images, such as photographs of wounds or skin conditions, and automatically generate descriptions and assessments. This can help improve the accuracy and consistency of image-based documentation and support more effective communication among healthcare professionals.

Predictive Analytics for Care Planning

AI-driven predictive analytics can be used to analyze historical nursing documentation and other patient data to identify patterns and trends that may inform future care planning.

For instance, AI algorithms could analyze past nursing notes to predict a patient's risk of developing complications or experiencing adverse events, supporting more proactive and personalized care planning.

Benefits of AI-Driven Nursing Documentation

The integration of AI into nursing documentation offers several benefits, including:

1. Improved efficiency
2. Enhanced accuracy and consistency
3. Reduced errors and omissions
4. Improved communication and collaboration

Improved Efficiency

One of the primary benefits of AI-driven nursing documentation is increased efficiency. By automating the generation, organization, and analysis of patient records, AI can help reduce the time and effort required for nursing documentation, freeing up nursing staff to focus on direct patient care.

Enhanced Accuracy and Consistency

AI-driven nursing documentation can improve the accuracy and consistency of patient records by standardizing the documentation process and reducing the potential for human error.

For instance, NLP and NLG technologies can help ensure that key information is accurately recorded and organized in a consistent format, facilitating more effective communication among healthcare professionals and improving the overall quality of patient records.

Reduced Errors and Omissions

AI-driven nursing documentation can help minimize the risk of errors and omissions in patient records by automating the documentation process and providing real-time validation and feedback.

For example, AI algorithms could analyze nursing notes in real-time to identify potential errors, such as incorrect medication dosages or missing information, and provide alerts to prompt nursing staff to review and correct the documentation.

Improved Communication and Collaboration

Effective communication and collaboration among healthcare professionals are critical for ensuring high-quality patient care. AI-driven nursing documentation can support more efficient and accurate communication by automating the generation and organization of patient records, making it easier for healthcare professionals to access and share information.

Challenges and Barriers to AI-Driven Nursing Documentation

Despite the promising potential of AI in nursing documentation, several challenges and barriers must be addressed for its successful implementation, including:

1. Data quality and availability
2. Integration with existing systems
3. Regulatory and ethical considerations
4. User acceptance and trust

Data Quality and Availability

The success of AI-driven nursing documentation is heavily dependent on the quality and availability of nursing and patient data. Ensuring that data is accurate, complete, and representative is critical for training AI algorithms and ensuring their reliable performance.

Integration with Existing Systems

Integrating AI-driven nursing documentationsolutions with existing healthcare systems and electronic health record (EHR) platforms can be challenging, requiring extensive collaboration and coordination among various stakeholders, including IT departments, nursing staff, and vendors.

Regulatory and Ethical Considerations

The use of AI in nursing documentation raises several regulatory and ethical considerations, such as patient privacy, data security, and algorithmic transparency. Ensuring compliance with relevant regulations and addressing ethical concerns is essential for the successful implementation of AI-driven nursing documentation.

User Acceptance and Trust

Achieving widespread adoption of AI-driven nursing documentation requires fostering user acceptance and trust among nursing staff and other healthcare professionals.

This involves addressing concerns related to potential job displacement, overreliance on technology, and the potential for AI algorithms to introduce new errors or biases into the documentation process.

Strategies for Successful Implementation

The successful implementation of AI-driven nursing documentation requires a comprehensive and strategic approach, including:

1. Investing in data infrastructure and quality
2. Engaging key stakeholders
3. Addressing regulatory and ethical considerations
4. Providing training and support

Investing in Data Infrastructure and Quality

Ensuring the availability and quality of nursing and patient data is a critical prerequisite for the successful implementation of AI-driven nursing documentation. This may involve investing in data infrastructure, standardizing data collection and documentation practices, and implementing data validation and quality control processes.

Engaging Key Stakeholders

Achieving buy-in and support from key stakeholders, such as nursing staff, IT departments, and hospital leadership, is essential for the successful implementation of AI-driven nursing documentation.

This may involve developing a shared vision and goals, involving stakeholders in the decision-making and implementation process, and fostering a culture of collaboration and innovation.

Addressing Regulatory and Ethical Considerations

Implementing AI-driven nursing documentation requires proactively addressing regulatory and ethical concerns, such as patient privacy, data security, and algorithmic transparency. This may involve engaging with regulatory authorities, conducting privacy and security risk assessments, and adopting transparent and accountable AI practices.

Providing Training and Support

Ensuring that nursing staff and other healthcare professionals have the necessary skills and knowledge to effectively use AI-driven nursing documentation tools is critical for their successful adoption. This may involve providing comprehensive training, ongoing support, and opportunities for feedback and continuous improvement.

Future Prospects and Research Directions

The application of AI in nursing documentation is a rapidly evolving field, with significant potential for further growth and innovation. Some promising future prospects and research directions include:

1. Expanding AI capabilities to cover a broader range of nursing tasks and specialties

2. Developing more advanced NLP and NLG techniques for improved documentation accuracy and efficiency

3. Exploring the potential for AI-driven nursing documentation to support clinical decision-making and care coordination

4. Investigating the impact of AI-driven nursing documentation on patient outcomes and healthcare costs

Conclusion

AI-driven nursing documentation holds significant promise for streamlining the documentation process, improving the quality of patient records, and supporting more efficient and accurate communication among healthcare professionals.

By addressing the challenges and barriers to implementation, such as data quality, integration, regulatory and ethical considerations, and user acceptance, healthcare organizations can successfully integrate AI-driven nursing documentation into their practice and realize its potential benefits.

As the field continues to evolve and mature, ongoing research and innovation will likely expand the capabilities of AI-driven nursing documentation and further enhance its impact on patient care and healthcare systems.

Furthermore, fostering a culture of collaboration, innovation, and continuous improvement will be essential for maximizing the potential of AI-driven nursing documentation and ensuring its long-term success in supporting high-quality patient care.

conclusion , AI-driven nursing documentation represents an exciting and transformative opportunity for healthcare organizations, with the potential to significantly improve the efficiency, accuracy, and quality of nursing documentation and support more effective communication and collaboration among healthcare professionals.

By embracing the potential of AI-driven nursing documentation and addressing the associated challenges and barriers, healthcare organizations can position themselves at the forefront of innovation and drive meaningful improvements in patient care and outcomes.

AI in Health Education and Training for Nursing: A Comprehensive Overview

Chapter 8: AI in Health Education and Training for Nursing: A Comprehensive Overview

Introduction

In recent years, artificial intelligence (AI) has emerged as a powerful tool for transforming various aspects of healthcare, including health education and training for nursing professionals. The integration of AI into nursing education can enhance the learning experience, personalize the training process, and improve the overall effectiveness of nursing education programs. This chapter will provide an in-depth overview of AI in health education and training for nursing, covering its applications, benefits, challenges, and future prospects.

The Role of AI in Health Education and Training for Nursing

AI has the potential to revolutionize nursing education and training by enabling more personalized, efficient, and engaging learning experiences. Key areas of AI application in nursing education and training include:

1. Adaptive learning systems

2. Virtual simulations and immersive technologies

3. AI-driven assessment and feedback

4. AI-powered educational resources

Adaptive Learning Systems

Adaptive learning systems use AI algorithms to analyze learners' performance and adapt the content and pacing of instruction to meet their individual needs. In the context of nursing education, adaptive learning systems can help create personalized learning pathways for students, ensuring that they receive the most relevant and effective instruction based on their unique strengths and weaknesses.

Virtual Simulations and Immersive Technologies

Virtual simulations and immersive technologies, such as virtual reality (VR) and augmented reality (AR), can be used in combination with AI to create realistic and interactive learning environments for nursing students.

These technologies can help nursing students develop clinical skills and decision-making abilities in a safe and controlled setting, enabling them to gain valuable experience and confidence before transitioning to real-world clinical practice.

AI-Driven Assessment and Feedback

AI-driven assessment and feedback tools can be used to evaluate nursing students' performance and provide targeted feedback to help them improve their skills and knowledge. For example, AI algorithms can analyze student responses to assessment tasks, identify areas of weakness, and generate personalized feedback to guide students' learning and development.

AI-Powered Educational Resources

AI can also be used to enhance the quality and accessibility of educational resources for nursing students. For instance, AI-powered search engines and recommendation systems can help students find relevant and high-quality learning materials, while AI-driven content analysis and summarization tools can help them process and retain information more effectively.

Benefits of AI Integration in Health Education and Training for Nursing

The integration of AI into nursing education and training offers several benefits, including:

1. Personalized learning experiences
2. Improved skill development and clinical decision-making
3. Enhanced access to educational resources

Personalized Learning Experiences

One of the primary benefits of AI-driven nursing education and training is the ability to create personalized learning experiences for students. By analyzing students' performance data and adapting the content and pacing of instruction to their individual needs, AI can help ensure that students receive the most effective and relevant learning experiences possible.

Improved Skill Development and Clinical Decision-Making

AI-driven simulations and immersive technologies can help nursing students develop their clinical skills and decision-making abilities in a safe and controlled environment.

This can lead to improved performance in real-world clinical settings, as students are better prepared to apply their knowledge and skills in practice.

Enhanced Access to Educational Resources

AI can help improve the accessibility and quality of educational resources for nursing students by facilitating the discovery of relevant and high-quality learning materials and enhancing the efficiency of content consumption and retention.

Challenges and Barriers to AI Integration in Nursing Education and Training

Despite its potential benefits, there are several challenges and barriers to the successful integration of AI in nursing education and training, including:

1. Data privacy and security concerns
2. Technical infrastructure and resource requirements
3. Teacher and student acceptance and trust

Data Privacy and Security Concerns

The use of AI in nursing education and training involves the collection, storage, and analysis of large amounts of student data, raising concerns about data privacy and security. Ensuring compliance with relevant regulations and addressing these concerns is crucial for the successful implementation of AI-driven education and training solutions.

Technical Infrastructure and Resource Requirements

Implementing AI-driven nursing education and training solutions requires significant investments in technical infrastructure and resources, such as hardware, software, and internet connectivit.

Ensuring that these resources are available and accessible to all students and educators is essential for the equitable implementation of AI-driven education and training programs.

Teacher and Student Acceptance and Trust

Achieving widespread adoption of AI-driven nursing education and training solutions requires fostering acceptance and trust among teachers and students. This involves addressing concerns related to potential job displacement, overreliance on technology, and the potential for AI algorithms to introduce new errors or biases into the education and training process.

Strategies for Successful Implementation

The successful implementation of AI-driven nursing education and training requires a comprehensive and strategic approach, including:

1. Addressing data privacy and security2. Ensuring equitable access to resources

3. Providing professional development opportunities

4. Fostering a culture of innovation and collaboration

Addressing Data Privacy and Security

To address data privacy and security concerns, nursing education institutions should work with experts to develop and implement robust data protection policies and practices. These policies should comply with relevant regulations and ensure the secure storage, transmission, and processing of student data.

Ensuring Equitable Access to Resources

Ensuring that all students and educators have access to the necessary technical infrastructure and resources is essential for the equitable implementation of AI-driven nursing education and training programs. Institutions should invest in upgrading their infrastructure and providing access to necessary hardware, software, and internet connectivity.

Providing Professional Development Opportunities

To help nursing educators and students successfully adopt and use AI-driven education and training solutions, institutions should provide professional development opportunities focused on the effective use of AI in nursing education. These opportunities could include workshops, webinars, and mentoring programs.

Fostering a Culture of Innovation and Collaboration

Promoting a culture of innovation and collaboration among nursing educators and students can help facilitate the successful integration of AI in nursing education and training. Institutions should encourage experimentation with new technologies and approaches, and provide opportunities for educators and students to collaborate on the development and implementation of AI-driven solutions.

Conclusion

AI has the potential to significantly enhance health education and training for nursing professionals, offering personalized learning experiences, improved skill development, and enhanced access to educational resources. However, to fully realize the benefits of AI in nursing education and training, it is crucial to address the challenges and barriers associated with its integration, such as data privacy and security concerns, technical infrastructure requirements, and teacher and student acceptance and trust. By adopting a strategic and collaborative approach, nursing education institutions can successfully implement AI-driven solutions that enhance the quality and effectiveness of nursing education and training, ultimately improving patient care and outcomes.

AI in Patient Care and Support: A Comprehensive Overview

Chapter 9: AI in Patient Care and Support: A Comprehensive Overview

Introduction

Artificial intelligence (AI) is transforming various aspects of healthcare, including patient care and support. AI-driven technologies have the potential to enhance patient care by improving diagnostics, personalizing treatment plans, and streamlining care delivery. This chapter will provide an in-depth overview of the role of AI in patient care and support, covering its applications, benefits, challenges, and future prospects in 20 pages.

The Role of AI in Patient Care and Support

AI-driven technologies can be applied in a range of patient care and support contexts, including:

1. Diagnostics and medical imaging
2. Personalized medicine and treatment planning
3. Remote monitoring and telemedicine
4. Support for healthcare professionals

Diagnostics and Medical Imaging

AI has shown promise in enhancing the accuracy and efficiency of diagnostics and medical imaging. AI algorithms can analyze complex medical images to identify abnormalities and support clinical decision-making.

Personalized Medicine and Treatment Planning

AI-driven technologies can analyze patient data to identify individualized treatment plans and optimize care delivery. This approach considers each patient's unique genetic, physiological, and lifestyle factors to tailor treatments for maximum efficacy.

Remote Monitoring and Telemedicine

AI can be utilized in remote monitoring and telemedicine applications to provide timely care and support to patients outside traditional healthcare settings. AI-driven tools can analyze data from wearable devices and other sensors to detect changes in patients' conditions and provide personalized feedback and recommendations.

Support for Healthcare Professionals

AI can assist healthcare professionals in their decision-making processes, providing evidence-based recommendations and reducing the likelihood of errors. AI-driven clinical decision support systems can help healthcare professionals to diagnose and treat patients more effectively.

Benefits of AI Integration in Patient Care and Support

The integration of AI-driven technologies into patient care and support offers several potential benefits, including:

1. Improved diagnostic accuracy
2. Personalized and optimized treatment plans
3. Enhanced care accessibility
4. Support for healthcare professionals and reduced errors

Improved Diagnostic Accuracy

AI-driven diagnostics and medical imaging tools can help healthcare providers identify diseases and conditions more accurately and efficiently. By analyzing complex medical images and patient data, AI algorithms can detect subtle abnormalities and enable earlier interventions.

Personalized and Optimized Treatment Plans

AI-driven personalized medicine and treatment planning can help healthcare providers tailor treatments to individual patients, optimizing care delivery and improving patient outcomes.

Enhanced Care Accessibility

Remote monitoring and telemedicine applications powered by AI can provide patients with access to care and support outside traditional healthcare settings. This can help bridge the gap for patients in rural or underserved areas and improve overall healthcare accessibility.

Support for Healthcare Professionals and Reduced Errors

AI-driven clinical decision support systems can help healthcare professionals make more informed decisions, reducing the likelihood of errors and improving patient care.

Challenges and Barriers to AI Integration in Patient Care and Support

Despite its potential benefits, there are several challenges and barriers to the successful integration of AI-driven technologies in patient care and support, including:

1. Data privacy and security concerns

2. Ethical considerations and algorithmic bias

3. Regulatory and legal issues

4. Healthcare professional acceptance and trust.

Data Privacy and Security Concerns

AI-driven patient care and support technologies rely on the collection, storage, and analysis of large amounts of patient data, raising concerns about data privacy and security. Ensuring compliance with relevant regulations and addressing these concerns is crucial for the successful implementation of AI-driven care solutions.

Ethical Considerations and Algorithmic Bias

Ethical considerations, such as ensuring that AI-driven technologies do not exacerbate existing healthcare disparities or introduce new biases, are essential for the responsible implementation of AI in patient care and support.

Regulatory and Legal Issues

Navigating the complex regulatory landscape surrounding AI-driven healthcare technologies is a significant challenge. Ensuring that AI-driven patient care and support tools meet relevant regulatory requirements and obtain necessary approvals is essential for their successful integration.

Healthcare Professional Acceptance and Trust

Achieving widespread adoption of AI-driven patient care and support technologies requires fostering acceptance and trust among healthcare professionals. This involves addressing concerns related to potential job displacement, overreliance on technology, and the potential for AI algorithms to introduce new errors or biases into the care process.

Strategies for Successful Implementation

The successful implementation of AI-driven patient care and support technologies requires a comprehensive and strategic approach, including:

1. Addressing data privacy and security
2. Ensuring ethical considerations are addressed
3. Navigating regulatory and legal issues
4. Fostering healthcare professional acceptance and trust.

Addressing Data Privacy and Security

To address data privacy and security concerns, healthcare institutions should work with experts to develop and implement robust data protection policies and practices. These policies should complywith relevant regulations and ensure that patient data is securely stored, transmitted, and analyzed.

Ensuring Ethical Considerations are Addressed

To address ethical considerations and prevent algorithmic bias, healthcare organizations should collaborate with multidisciplinary teams of experts, including ethicists, data scientists, and clinicians. These teams can help ensure that AI-driven technologies are designed and implemented responsibly and equitably.

Navigating Regulatory and Legal Issues

Navigating the complex regulatory landscape requires collaboration between healthcare organizations, technology developers, and regulatory authorities. By working together, these stakeholders can help ensure that AI-driven patient care and support tools meet necessary requirements and obtain the necessary approvals for implementation.

Fostering Healthcare Professional Acceptance and Trust

To build acceptance and trust among healthcare professionals, organizations should prioritize education and training on AI-driven technologies. This includes providing opportunities for healthcare professionals to learn about the benefits, risks, and limitations of AI-driven tools and offering hands-on experience with these technologies.

Examples of AI-driven Patient Care and Support Technologies

There are numerous examples of AI-driven patient care and support technologies currently in use or under development, including:

1. AI-driven diagnostics and medical imaging tools
2. AI-driven personalized medicine and treatment planning solutions
3. Remote monitoring and telemedicine applications
4. AI-driven clinical decision support systems

AI-driven Diagnostics and Medical Imaging Tools

AI-driven diagnostics and medical imaging tools include solutions for detecting and diagnosing various diseases and conditions. Examples include AI algorithms for analyzing chest X-rays to identify pneumonia and deep learning models for diagnosing diabetic retinopathy from retinal images.

AI-driven Personalized Medicine and Treatment Planning Solutions

AI-driven personalized medicine and treatment planning solutions include tools for analyzing genomic data to identify targeted therapies for cancer patients and algorithms capable of predicting patient responses to specific medications based on their unique genetic profiles.

Remote Monitoring and Telemedicine Applications

Remote monitoring and telemedicine applications include AI-driven tools for analyzing data from wearable devices and other sensors to detect changes in patients' conditions and provide personalized feedback and recommendations. These technologies can help patients manage chronic conditions and reduce the need for in-person visits.

AI-driven Clinical Decision Support Systems

AI-driven clinical decision support systems include tools that analyze patient data and provide healthcare professionals with evidence-based recommendations for diagnosis and treatment. These systems can help to reduce errors and improve patient outcomes by providing healthcare professionals with timely and relevant information.

Conclusion

AI-driven patient care and support technologies have the potential to transform healthcare, improving diagnostic accuracy, personalizing treatment plans, and streamlining care delivery. By addressing challenges related to data privacy, ethical considerations, regulatory issues, and healthcare professional acceptance, healthcare organizations can successfully integrate AI-driven tools into their care processes and improve patient outcomes. As AI continues to advance, the potential for further innovations and improvements in patient care and support is vast, promising a brighter future for healthcare.

AI Ethical Considerations: A Comprehensive Overview

Chapter 10: AI Ethical Considerations: A Comprehensive Overview

Introduction

Artificial intelligence (AI) holds tremendous potential for transforming various aspects of society, including healthcare, finance, education, and more. However, as AI technologies become more sophisticated and integrated into our daily lives, it is essential to address the ethical considerations that emerge. This chapter will provide a comprehensive overview of AI ethical considerations, covering topics such as data privacy, algorithmic bias, transparency, accountability, the impact on employment, and developing ethical AI frameworks.

Key Ethical Considerations in AI

The integration of AI technologies into various sectors raises several ethical considerations, including:

1. Data privacy and security
2. Algorithmic bias and fairness
3. Transparency and explainability
4. Accountability and responsibility
5. Impact on employment
6. Autonomous decision-making.

Data Privacy and Security

AI systems often rely on large datasets to learn and make decisions. The collection, storage, and analysis of personal data raise concerns about data privacy and security. Ensuring that AI systems handle personal data responsibly, comply with relevant regulations, and protect against unauthorized access is vital.

Algorithmic Bias and Fairness

AI algorithms can perpetuate or exacerbate existing biases if they are trained on biased data or developed without considering fairness. Addressing algorithmic bias is crucial for ensuring that AI technologies do not discriminate against certain groups or individuals and contribute to a just and equitable society.

Transparency and Explainability

AI systems can be complex and opaque, making it challenging to understand how they make decisions. Ensuring that AI systems are transparent and explainable is essential for fostering trust, enabling effective oversight, and facilitating informed decision-making by users and other stakeholders.

Accountability and Responsibility

As AI systems become more autonomous, determining accountability and responsibility for their actions becomes more complex. It is essential to establish clear guidelines and frameworks for assigning accountability and responsibility for AI-driven decisions and outcomes.

Impact on Employment

AI technologies have the potential to automate various tasks, which can lead to job displacement and changes in the labor market. Addressing the ethical implications of AI's impact on employment, including ensuring that AI-driven automation benefits society more broadly and does not exacerbate existing inequalities, is crucial.

Autonomous Decision-Making

AI systems capable of making autonomous decisions raise ethical concerns related to human agency and moral responsibility. Developing guidelines and frameworks for the ethical use of autonomous AI systems is essential for ensuring that these technologies respect human values and rights.

Developing Ethical AI Frameworks

To address the ethical considerations discussed above, it is essential to develop comprehensive ethical AI frameworks. These frameworks should provide guidance on best practices for AI development, deployment, and governance, helping stakeholders navigate the complex ethical landscape surrounding AI technologies.

Multidisciplinary Approach

Developing ethical AI frameworks requires a multidisciplinary approach, bringing together experts from various fields, including computer science, ethics, social sciences, law, and more. This collaborative approach helps ensure that ethical AI frameworks are comprehensive, well-informed, and capable of addressing the diverse range of ethical considerations arising from AI technologies.

Inclusive Stakeholder Engagement

In addition to involving experts from various disciplines, developing ethical AI frameworks should involve engaging with a wide range of stakeholders, including AI developers, users, policymakers, and the public. Inclusive stakeholder engagement can help ensure that ethical AI frameworks are responsive to the needs and concerns of different groups and that the benefits and risks of AI technologies are distributed equitably.

Iterative and Adaptive Process

Developing ethical AI frameworks should be an iterative and adaptive process, responding to the rapid evolution of AI technologies and the emergence of new ethical considerations. Regularly revisiting and updating ethical AI frameworks can help ensure that they remain relevant and effective in addressing the ethical challenges posed by AI.

Examples of Ethical AI Frameworks and Guidelines

Several organizations and initiatives have developed ethical AI frameworks and guidelines, including:

1. The European Commission's Ethics Guidelines for Trustworthy AI
2. The IEEE's Ethically Aligned Design
3. The Partnership on AI's Tenets
4. The Asilomar AI Principles

The European Commission's Ethics Guidelines for Trustworthy AI

The European Commission's Ethics Guidelines for Trustworthy AI outline seven key requirements for achieving trustworthy AI, including human agency and oversight, technical robustness and safety, privacy and data governance, transparency, fairness, societal and environmental well-being, and accountability.

The IEEE's Ethically Aligned Design

The IEEE's Ethically Aligned Design initiative provides a set of ethical principles and recommendations for the development and use of AI and autonomous systems, addressing topics such as human rights, data privacy, transparency, and accountability.

The Partnership on AI's Tenets

The Partnership on AI, amulti-stakeholder initiative that includes leading technology companies, academics, and civil society organizations, has developed a set of tenets aimed at guiding the development and deployment of AI technologies. The tenets focus on ensuring AI benefits all, promoting long-term safety, technical leadership, and cooperative orientation.

The Asilomar AI Principles

The Asilomar AI Principles, developed during the Asilomar Conference on Beneficial AI, outline 23 principles for guiding the development of AI technologies. These principles emphasize the importance of broadly distributed benefits, long-term safety, transparent research, and cooperation among researchers and developers.

Conclusion

As AI technologies become increasingly integrated into various aspects of society, addressing the ethical considerations that arise is crucial. By understanding and addressing concerns related to data privacy, algorithmic bias, transparency, accountability, the impact on employment, and autonomous decision-making, we can ensure that AI technologies are developed and deployed responsibly and ethically. Developing comprehensive ethical AI frameworks, engaging with diverse stakeholders, and adopting a multidisciplinary and adaptive approach are essential steps towards achieving this goal. By doing so, we can harness the potential of AI to benefit society while mitigating its potential risks and harms.

Future Prospects for Nursing in the Artificial Intelligence

Chapter 8: Future Prospects for Nursing in the Artificial Intelligence

Introduction

Artificial intelligence (AI) is rapidly transforming various sectors, including healthcare. As AI technologies continue to advance and become more integrated into healthcare systems, the nursing profession is poised to undergo significant changes. This chapter will explore the future prospects for nursing in the AI era, discussing the potential benefits and challenges associated with AI adoption, as well as the evolving roles and responsibilities of nurses.

AI in Nursing: Potential Benefits

AI technologies have the potential to revolutionize nursing by:

1. Enhancing decision-making and clinical judgment
2. Automating routine tasks and improving efficiency
3. Facilitating personalized patient care
4. Improving patient monitoring and early detection

Enhancing Decision-Making and Clinical Judgment

AI-powered tools and applications can help nurses make more informed decisions by providing real-time access to patient data, clinical guidelines, and evidence-based recommendations. This enhanced decision-making support can improve patient outcomes, reduce errors, and enable nurses to provide higher quality care.

Automating Routine Tasks and Improving Efficiency

AI technologies can automate various routine tasks, such as medication administration, documentation, and patient scheduling, freeing up nurses to focus on more complex and patient-centered aspects of care. This increased efficiency can lead to improved patient experiences and reduced nurse workload and burnout.

Facilitating Personalized Patient Care

AI can help nurses deliver personalized care by analyzing patient data and generating individualized treatment recommendations. By tailoring care to each patient's unique needs, nurses can improve patient outcomes and satisfaction.

Improving Patient Monitoring and Early Detection

AI-powered monitoring systems can enable continuous, real-time monitoring of patients, detecting subtle changes in their conditions and alerting nurses to potential issues. This early detection can help prevent complications and enable timely interventions, ultimately improving patient outcomes.

Challenges and Considerations in AI Adoption

While AI holds tremendous potential for transforming nursing, it also raises several challenges and considerations, including:

1. Data privacy and security
2. Algorithmic bias and fairness
3. Technology acceptance and adoption
4. Education and training
5. Ethical considerations

Data Privacy and Security

The integration of AI technologies into nursing practice requires careful attention to data privacy and security, ensuring that patient information is protected and used responsibly. Compliance with relevant regulations, such as HIPAA in the United States, and implementing robust security measures are essential for safeguarding patient data.

Algorithmic Bias and Fairness

AI systems can perpetuate existing biases and inequities if not designed and trained carefully. Ensuring that AI tools used in nursing are free from bias and fair to all patients is crucial for maintaining trust and providing equitable care.

Technology Acceptance and Adoption

Nurses' acceptance and adoption of AI technologies are critical for realizing their potential benefits. Addressing concerns about job displacement, fostering a culture of innovation, and providing adequate support are essential for facilitating the successful integration of AI into nursing practice.

Education and Training

As AI technologies become more prevalent in nursing, it is essential to equip nurses with the knowledge and skills needed to use these tools effectively. This includes incorporating AI education into nursing curricula and providing ongoing training and professional development opportunities.

Ethical Considerations

AI's integration into nursing practice raises several ethical considerations, such as the potential for dehumanization of care, loss of human touch, and concerns about the autonomy of AI-powered tools. Addressing these ethical concerns is essential for ensuring that AI technologies are used responsibly and align with nursing's core values and principles.

Evolving Roles and Responsibilities of Nurses

As AI becomes more integrated into healthcare systems, the roles and responsibilities of nurses are likely to evolve. Key areas of change may include:

1. Expanding scope of practice
2. Greater emphasis on care coordination
3. Increased focus on patient advocacy and education

Expanding Scope of Practice

With AI technologies taking on more routine tasks, nurses may see their scope of practice expand, allowing them to focus on higher-level clinical activities, decision-making, and more complex patient care.

Greater Emphasis on Care Coordination

As AI streamlines various aspects of nursing, nurses may increasingly take on care coordination roles, ensuring that patients receive well-integrated, comprehensive care across the healthcare continuum.

Increased Focus on Patient Advocacy and Education

As patients become more involved in their care and AI technologies play a more prominent role, nurses may take on a more significant role in patient advocacy and education, helping patients understand and navigate the increasingly complex healthcare landscape.

Conclusion

The future prospects for nursing in the AI era are characterized by both exciting opportunities and significant challenges. While AI technologies have the potential to revolutionize nursing practice, their successful integration requires careful attention to data privacy, algorithmic bias, technology acceptance, education, and ethical considerations. Asthe roles and responsibilities of nurses evolve, it is essential to prepare the nursing workforce for these changes through education, training, and ongoing professional development.

By embracing AI technologies and cultivating a culture of innovation, the nursing profession can capitalize on the opportunities presented by the AI era. This includes enhancing decision-making, improving efficiency, facilitating personalized care, and promoting better patient outcomes. However, it is crucial to ensure that the adoption of AI technologies aligns with nursing's core values and principles, maintaining the focus on compassionate, patient-centered care.

Ultimately, the successful integration of AI into nursing practice will depend on the ability of nurses, educators, policymakers, and other stakeholders to navigate the challenges and opportunities presented by these transformative technologies. By working together, we can ensure that the future of nursing is one where AI technologies complement and enhance the essential role of nurses in healthcare.

By Ahmed Ragab Ali Abdelghany **MSYTR**